My Dash Diet Cookbook

Balanced, Simple and delicious Recipes for Your
Health

Natalie Puckett

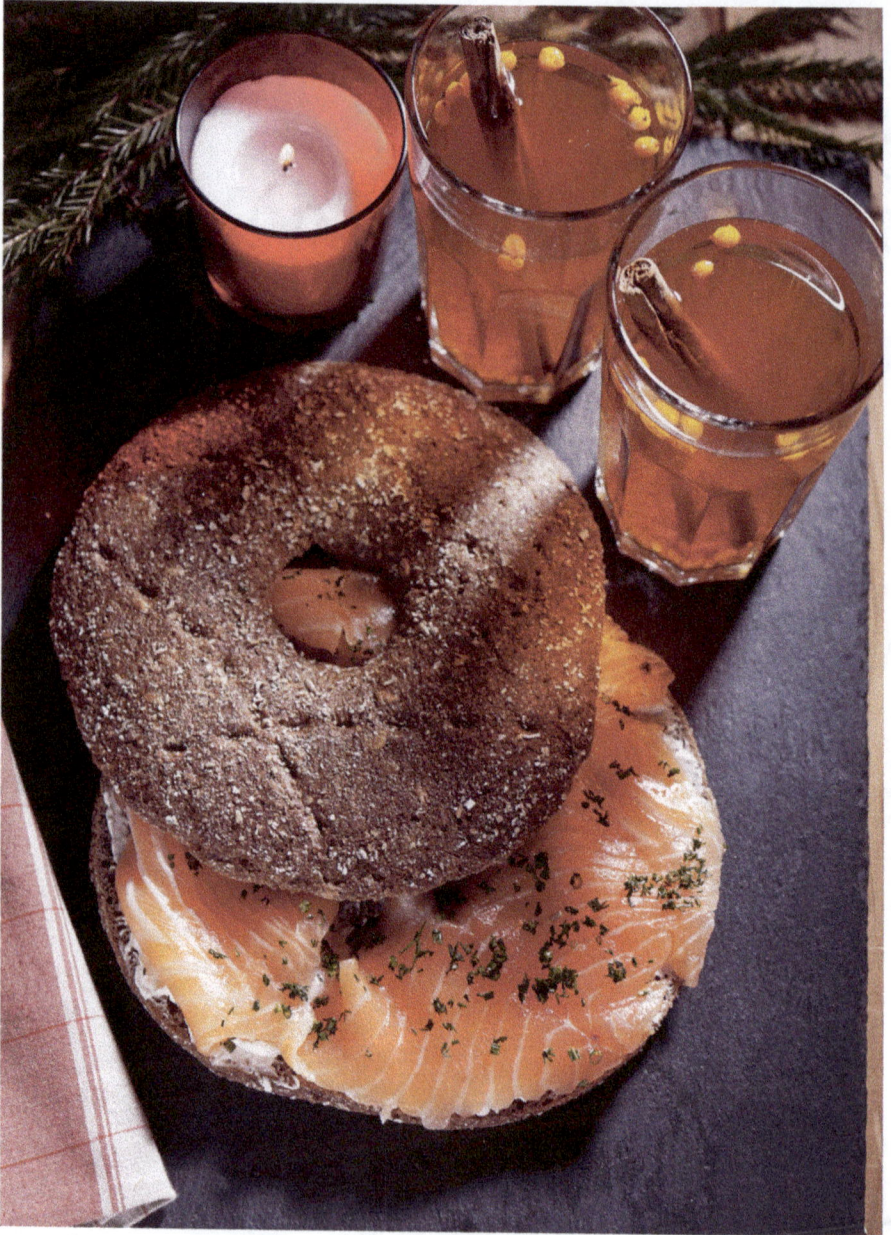

Table of Contents

Cinnamon Salmon

Serving: 4

Prep Time: 10 minutes

Cook Time: 10 minutes

Ingredients:

2 salmon fillets, boneless and skin on

Pepper to taste

1 tablespoon cinnamon powder

1 tablespoon organic olive oil

How To:

1.   Take a pan and place it over medium heat, add oil and let it heat up.

2.   Add pepper, cinnamon and stir.

3.   Add salmon, skin side up and cook for five minutes on each side.

4.   Divide between plates and serve.

5.   Enjoy!

Nutrition (Per Serving)

Calories: 220

Fat: 8g

Carbohydrates: 11g

Protein: 8g

Scallop and Strawberry Mix

Serving: 4

Prep Time: 10 minutes

Cook Time: 6 minutes

Ingredients:

ounces scallops

½ cup Pico De Gallo

½ cup strawberries, chopped

1 tablespoon lime juice

Pepper to taste

How To:

1.   Take a pan and place it over medium heat, add scallops and cook for 3 minutes on each side.

2.   Remove heat.

3.   Take a bowl and add strawberries, juice , Pico De Gallo, scallops, pepper and toss well.

4.   Serve and enjoy!

Nutrition (Per Serving)

Calories: 169

Fat: 2g

Carbohydrates: 8g

Protein: 13g

Salmon and Orange Dish

Serving: 4

Prep Time: 10 minutes

Cook Time: 15 minutes

Ingredients:

salmon fillets

cup orange juice

tablespoons arrowroot and water mixture 1 teaspoon orange peel, grated 1 teaspoon black pepper

How To:

1.   Add the listed ingredients to your pot.

2.   Lock the lid and cook on high for 12 minutes.

3.   Release the pressure naturally.

4.   Serve and enjoy!

Nutrition (Per Serving)

Calories:583

Fat: 20g

Carbohydrates: 71g

Protein: 33g

Mesmerizing Coconut Haddock

Serving: 3

Prep Time: 10 minutes

Cook Time: 12 minutes

Ingredients:

Haddock fillets, 5 ounces each, boneless 2 tablespoons coconut oil, melted

1 cup coconut, shredded and unsweetened

¼ cup hazelnuts, ground Sunflower seeds to taste

How To:

1.   Pre-heat your oven to 400 degrees F.

2.   Line a baking sheet with parchment paper.

3.   Keep it on the side.

4.   Pat fish fillets with towel and season with sunflower seeds.

5.   Take a bowl and stir in hazelnuts and shredded coconut.

6.   Drag fish fillets through the coconut mix until each side are coated well.

7.   Transfer to baking dish.

8.   Brush with copra oil .

9.   Bake for about 12 minutes until flaky.

10.   Serve and enjoy!

Nutrition (Per Serving)

Calories: 299

Fat: 24g

Carbohydrates: 1g

Protein: 20g

Asparagus and Lemon Salmon

Dish

Serving: 3

Prep Time: 5 minutes

Cook Time: 15 minutes

Ingredients:

2 salmon fillets, 6 ounces each, skin on Sunflower seeds to taste

1-pound asparagus, trimmed 2 cloves garlic, minced tablespoons almond butter ¼ cup cashew cheese

How To:

Pre-heat your oven to 400 degrees F.

Line a baking sheet with oil.

Take a kitchen towel and pat your salmon dry, season as needed.

1.   Put salmon onto the baking sheet and arrange asparagus around it.

2.   Place a pan over medium heat and melt almond butter.

3.   Add garlic and cook for 3 minutes until garlic browns slightly.

4.   Drizzle sauce over salmon.

5.   Sprinkle salmon with cheese and bake for 12 minutes until salmon looks cooked all the way and is flaky.

6.   Serve and enjoy!

Nutrition (Per Serving)

Calories: 434

Fat: 26g

Carbohydrates: 6g

Protein: 42g

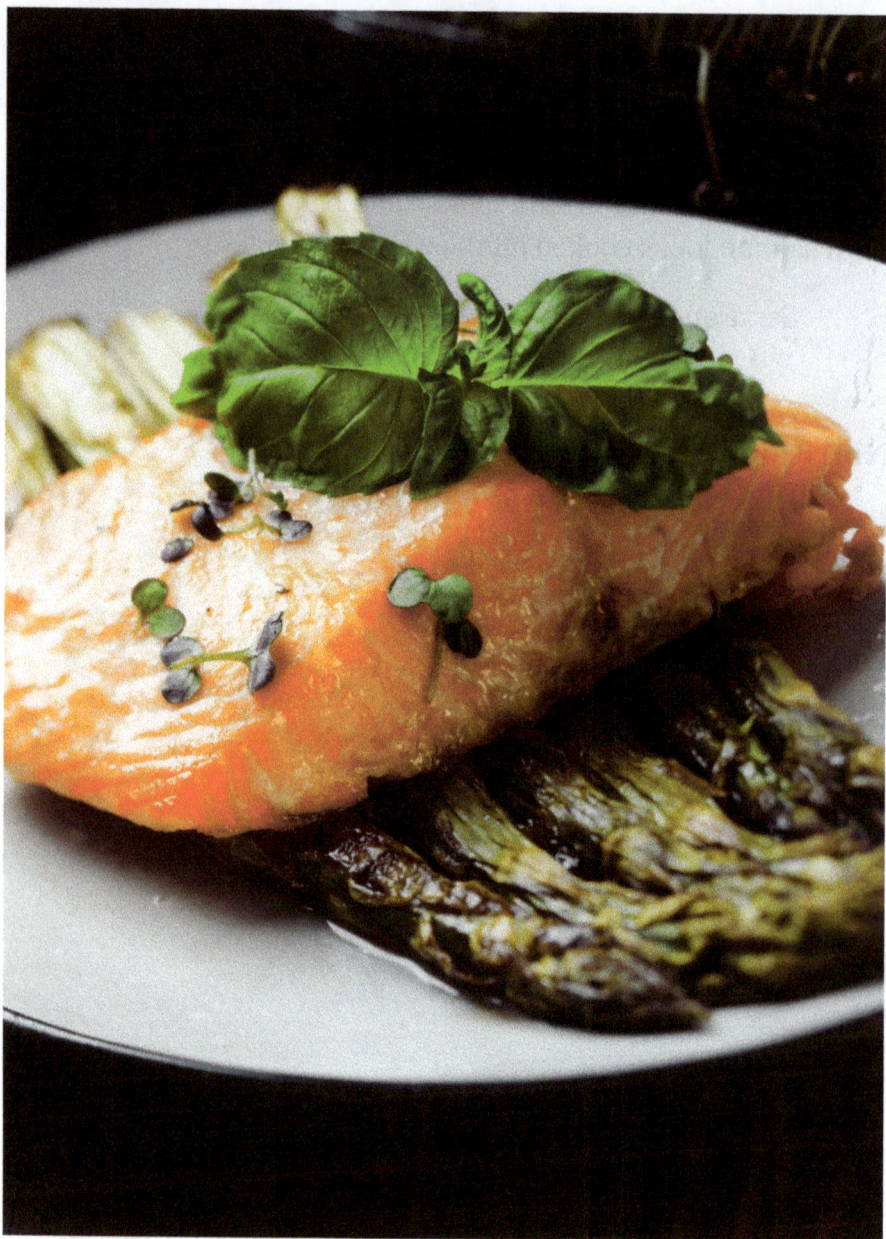

Lamb Curry with Tomatoes And Spinach

Prep time: 10 minutes

Cook time: 12 minutes

Servings: 4

Ingredients

Olive oil – 1 tsp

Lean boneless lamb – 1 pound, sliced thinly Onion – 1, chopped

Garlic – 3 cloves, minced Red bell pepper – 1, chopped Salt-free tomato paste – 2 Tbsp.

Salt-free curry powder – 1 Tbsp.

No-salt-added diced tomatoes – 1(15-ounce) can

Fresh baby spinach – 10 ounces

Low-sodium beef or vegetable broth - ½ cup

Red wine – ¼ cup

Chopped fresh cilantro – ¼ cup Ground black pepper to taste

Method

1.   Heat the oil in a pan.

2.   Add lamb and brown both sides, about 2 minutes.

3.   Add garlic, onion, and bell pepper. Stir-fry for 2 minutes. Stir in the curry powder and tomato paste.

4.   Add the tomatoes with juice, spinach, broth, and wine and stir to mix.

5.   Stir-fry for 3 to 4 minutes and lamb has cooked through.

6.   Remove from heat. Season with pepper and stir in cilantro.

7.   Serve.

Nutritional Facts Per Serving

Calories: 238

Fat: 7g

Carb: 14g

Protein: 27g

Sodium 167mg

Pomegranate-Marinated Leg of Lamb

Prep time: 10 minutes

Cook time: 20 minutes

Servings: 6

Ingredients

For the marinate

Bottled pomegranate juice - ½ cup

Hearty red wine – ½ cup

Ground cumin - 1 tsp.

Dried oregano – 1 tsp.

Crushed hot red pepper – ½ tsp.

Garlic – 3 cloves, minced

For the lamb

Boneless leg of lamb – 1 ¾ pound, butterflied and fat trimmed

Kosher salt – ½ tsp.

Olive oil spray

Method

1.   To make the marinade, whisk everything in a bowl and transfer to a zippered plastic bag.

2.   To prepare the lamb: add the lamb to the bag, press out the air, and close the bag. Marinate for 1 hour in the refrigerator.

3.   Preheat the broiler (8 inches from the source of heat).

4.   Remove the lamb from the marinade, blot with paper towels, but do not dry completely.

5.   Season with salt. Spray the broiler rack with oil.

6.   Place the lamb on the rack and broil, turning occasionally, about 20 minutes, or until lamb is browned and reaches 130F.

7.   Remove from heat, slice and serve with carving juices on top.

Nutritional Facts Per Serving

Calories: 273

Fat: 15g

Carb: 0g

Protein: 31g

Sodium 219mg

Beef Fajitas with Peppers

Prep time: 10 minutes

Cook time: 12 minutes

Servings: 6

Ingredients

Olive oil – 2 tsp. plus more for the spray

Sirloin steak – 1 pound, cut into bite-size pieces

Red bell pepper – 1, chopped

Green bell pepper – 1, chopped

Red onion – 1, chopped

Garlic - 2 cloves, minced

DASH friendly Mexican seasoning – 1 Tbsp. (or any seasoning without salt)

Boston lettuce leaves – 12 for serving Lime wedges or corn tortillas for serving

Method

Heat oil in a skillet.

Add half of the sirloin and cook until browned on both sides, about 2 minutes. Transfer to a plate.

Then repeat with the remaining sirloin.

Heat the 2 tsp. oil in the skillet.

Add onion, bell peppers, and garlic, cook and stir for 7 minutes or until tender.

Stir in the beef with any juices and the seasoning. Transfer to a plate.

Fill lettuce lead with beef mixture and drizzle lime juice on top.

Roll up and serve.

Nutritional Facts Per Serving

Calories: 231

Fat: 12g

Carb: 6g

Protein: 24g

Sodium 59mg

Pork Medallions with Herbs De Provence

Prep time: 5 minutes

Cook time: 10 minutes

Servings: 2

Ingredients

Pork tenderloin – 8 ounces, cut into 6 pieces (crosswise)

Ground black pepper to taste Herbs de Provence – ½ tsp. Dry white wine – ¼ cup

Method

1.   Season the pork with black pepper.

2.   Place the pork between waxed paper sheets and roll with a rolling pin until about ¼ inch thick.

3.   Cook the pork in a pan for 2 to 3 minutes on each side.

4.   Remove from heat and season with the herb.

5.   Place the pork on plates and keep warm.

6.   Cook the wine in the pan until boiling. Scrape to get the brown bits from the bottom.

7.   Serve pork with the sauce.

Nutritional Facts Per Serving

Calories: 120

Fat: 2g

Carb: 1g

Protein: 24g

Sodium 62mg

Ravaging Blueberry Muffin

Serving: 4

Prep Time: 10 minutes

Cook Time: 30 minutes

Ingredients:

1 cup almond flour

Pinch of sunflower seeds

1/8 teaspoon baking soda

1 whole egg

2 tablespoons coconut oil, melted

½ cup coconut almond milk

¼ cup fresh blueberries

How To:

1.   Pre-heat your oven to 350 degrees F.

2.   Line a muffin tin with paper muffin cups.

3.   Add almond flour, sunflower seeds, baking soda to a bowl and mix, keep it on the side.

4. Take another bowl and add egg, coconut oil, coconut almond milk and mix.

5. Add mix to flour mix and gently combine until incorporated.

6. Mix in blueberries and fill the cupcakes tins with batter.

7. Bake for 20-25 minutes.

8. Enjoy!

Nutrition (Per Serving)

Calories: 167

Fat: 15g

Carbohydrates: 2.1g

Protein: 5.2g

The Coconut Loaf

Serving: 4

Prep Time: 15 minutes

Cook Time: 40 minutes

Ingredients:

1 ½ tablespoons coconut flour

¼ teaspoon baking powder

1/8 teaspoon sunflower seeds

1 tablespoons coconut oil, melted

1 whole egg

How To:

1.   Pre-heat your oven to 350 degrees F.

2.   Add coconut flour, baking powder, sunflower seeds.

3.   Add coconut oil, eggs and stir well until mixed.

4.   Leave batter for several minutes.

5.   Pour half batter onto baking pan.

6.   Spread it to form a circle, repeat with remaining batter.

7.   Bake in oven for 10 minutes.

8.   Once you have a golden-brown texture, let it cool and serve.

9.   Enjoy!

Nutrition (Per Serving)

Calories: 297

Fat: 14g

Carbohydrates: 15g

Protein: 15g

Fresh Figs with Walnuts and Ricotta

Serving: 4

Prep Time: 5 minutes

Cook Time: 2-3 minutes

Ingredients:

8 dried figs, halved

¼ cup ricotta cheese

16 walnuts, halved

1 tablespoon honey

How To:

1.   Take a skillet and place it over medium heat, add walnuts and toast for 2 minutes.

2.   Top figs with cheese and walnuts.

3.   Drizzle honey on top.

4.   Enjoy!

Nutrition (Per Serving)

Calories: 142

Fat: 8g

Carbohydrates:10g

Protein:4g

Authentic Medjool Date Truffles

Serving: 4

Prep Time: 10-15 minutes

Cook Time: Nil

Ingredients:

2 tablespoons peanut oil

½ cup popcorn kernels

1/3 cup peanuts, chopped

1/3 cup peanut almond butter

¼ cup wildflower honey

How To:

1.   Take a pot and add popcorn kernels, peanut oil.

2.   Place it over medium heat and shake the pot gently until all corn has popped.

3.   Take a saucepan and add honey, gently simmer for 2-3 minutes.

4.   Add peanut almond butter and stir.

5.   Coat popcorn with the mixture and enjoy!

Nutrition (Per Serving)

Calories: 430

Fat: 20g

Carbohydrates: 56g

Protein 9g

Tasty Mediterranean Peanut

Almond butter Popcorns

Serving: 4

Prep Time: 5 minutes + 20 minutes chill time

Cook Time: 2-3 minutes

Ingredients:

3 cups Medjool dates, chopped

12 ounces brewed coffee 1 cup pecans, chopped ½ cup coconut, shredded ½ cup cocoa powder

How To:

1.   Soak dates in warm coffee for 5 minutes.

2.   Remove dates from coffee and mash them, making a fine smooth mixture.

3.   Stir in remaining ingredients (except cocoa powder) and form small balls out of the mixture.

4.   Coat with cocoa powder, serve and enjoy!

Nutrition (Per Serving)

Calories: 265

Fat: 12g

Carbohydrates: 43g

Protein 3g

One Minute Muffin

Serving: 2

Prep Time: 5 minutes

Cooking Time: 1 minute

Ingredients:

Coconut oil for grease

2 teaspoons coconut flour

1 pinch baking soda

1 pinch sunflower seed

1 whole egg

How To:

1. Grease ramekin dish with coconut oil and keep it on the side.

2. Add ingredients to a bowl and combine until no lumps.

3. Pour batter into ramekin.

4. Microwave for 1 minute on HIGH.

5. Slice in half and serve.

6.   Enjoy!

Nutrition (Per Serving)

Total Carbs: 5.4

Fiber: 2g

Protein: 7.3g

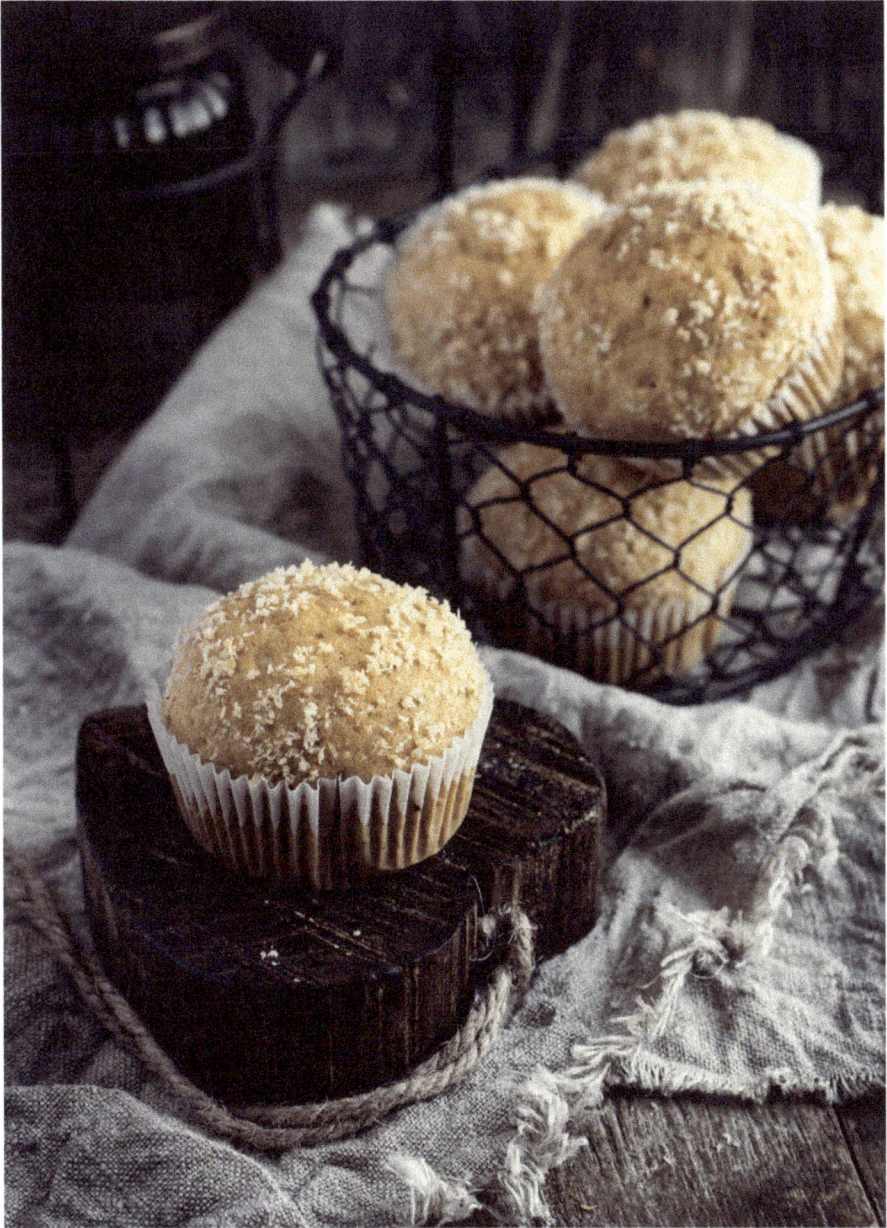

Hearty Almond Bread

Serving: 8

Prep Time: 15 minutes

Cook Time: 60 minutes

Ingredients:

3 cups almond flour

1 teaspoon baking soda

2 teaspoons baking powder

¼ teaspoon sunflower seeds

¼ cup almond milk

½ cup + 2 tablespoons olive oil

3 whole eggs

How To:

1.   Pre-heat your oven to 300 degrees F.

2.   Take a 9x5 inch loaf pan and grease, keep it on the side.

3.   Add listed ingredients to a bowl and pour the batter into the loaf pan.

4.   Bake for 60 minutes.

5.   Once baked, remove from oven and let it cool.

6.   Slice and serve!

Nutrition (Per Serving)

Calories: 277

Fat: 21g

Carbohydrates: 7g

Protein: 10g

Refreshing Mango and Pear Smoothie

Serving: 1

Prep Time: 10 minutes

Cook Time: Nil

Ingredients:

1 ripe mango, cored and chopped

½ mango, peeled, pitted and chopped

1 cup kale, chopped

½ cup plain Greek yogurt

2 ice cubes

How To:

1.   Add pear, mango, yogurt, kale, and mango to a blender and puree.

2.   Add ice and blend until you have a smooth texture.

3.   Serve and enjoy!

Nutrition (Per Serving)

Calories: 293

Fat: 8g

Carbohydrates: 53g

Protein: 8g

Coconut and Hazelnut Chilled Glass

Serving: 1

Prep Time: 10 minutes

Ingredients:

½ cup coconut almond milk

¼ cup hazelnuts, chopped

1 ½ cups water

1 pack stevia

How To:

1. Add listed ingredients to blender.

2. Blend until you have a smooth and creamy texture.

3. Serve chilled and enjoy!

Nutrition (Per Serving)

Calories: 457

Fat: 46g

Carbohydrates: 12g

Protein: 7g

The Mocha Shake

Serving: 1

Prep Time: 10 minutes

Ingredients:

1 cup whole almond milk

2 tablespoons cocoa powder2 packs stevia

1 cup brewed coffee, chilled

1 tablespoon coconut oil

How To:

1.   Add listed ingredients to blender.

2.   Blend until you have a smooth and creamy texture.

3.   Serve chilled and enjoy!

Nutrition (Per Serving)

Calories: 293

Fat: 23g

Carbohydrates: 19g

Protein: 10g

Cinnamon Chiller

Serving: 1

Prep Time: 10 minutes

Ingredients:

1 cup unsweetened almond milk

2 tablespoons vanilla protein powder

½ teaspoon cinnamon

¼ teaspoon vanilla extract

1 tablespoon chia seeds

1 cup ice cubs

How To:

1.   Add listed ingredients to blender.

2.   Blend until you have a smooth and creamy texture.

3.   Serve chilled and enjoy!

Nutrition (Per Serving)

Calories: 145

Fat: 4g

Carbohydrates: 1.6g

Protein: 0.6g

Hearty Alkaline Strawberry Summer Deluxe

Serving: 2

Prep Time: 5 minutes

Ingredients:

½ cup organic strawberries/blueberries

Half a banana

2 cups coconut water ½ inch ginger

Juice of 2 grapefruits

How To:

1. Add all the listed ingredients to your blender.

2. Blend until smooth.

3. Add a few ice cubes and serve the smoothie.

4. Enjoy!

Nutrition (Per Serving)

Calories: 200

Fat: 10g

Carbohydrates: 14g

Protein 2g

Mesmerizing Brussels and Pistachios

Serving: 4

Prep Time: 15 minutes

Cook Time: 15 minutes

Ingredients:

1-pound Brussels sprouts, tough bottom trimmed and halved lengthwise

1 tablespoon extra-virgin olive oil

Sunflower seeds and pepper as needed

½ cup roasted pistachios, chopped Juice of ½ lemon

How To:

1.   Pre-heat your oven to 400 degrees F.

2.   Line a baking sheet with aluminum foil and keep it on the side.

3.   Take a large bowl and add Brussels sprouts with olive oil and coat well.

4.　　Season sea sunflower seeds, pepper, spread veggies evenly on sheet.

5.　　Bake for 15 minutes until lightly caramelized.

6.　　Remove from oven and transfer to a serving bowl.

7.　　Toss with pistachios and lemon juice.

8.　　Serve warm and enjoy!

Nutrition (Per Serving)

Calories: 126

Fat: 7g

Carbohydrates: 14g

Protein: 6g

Brussels's Fever

Serving: 4

Prep Time: 10 minutes

Cook Time: 20 minutes

Ingredients:

2 tablespoons olive oil

1 yellow onion, chopped

2 pounds Brussels sprouts, trimmed and halved

4 cups vegetable stock

¼ cup coconut cream

How To:

1.   Take a pot and place it over medium heat.

2.   Add oil and let it heat up.

3.   Add onion and stir-cook for 3 minutes.

4.   Add Brussels sprouts and stir, cook for 2 minutes.

5.   Add stock and black pepper, stir and bring to a simmer.

6.   Cook for 20 minutes more.

7.   Use an immersion blender to make the soup creamy.

8.   Add coconut cream and stir well.

9.   Ladle into soup bowls and serve.

10.   Enjoy!

Nutrition (Per Serving)

Calories: 200

Fat: 11g

Carbohydrates: 6g

Protein: 11g

Hearty Garlic and Kale Platter

Serving: 4

Prep Time: 5 minutes

Cook Time: 10 minutes

Ingredients:

1 bunch kale

2 tablespoons olive oil

4 garlic cloves, minced

How To:

1.   Carefully tear the kale into bite sized portions, making sure to remove the stem.

2.   Discard the stems.

3.   Take a large sized pot and place it over medium heat.

4.   Add olive oil and let the oil heat up.

5.   Add garlic and stir for 2 minutes.

6.   Add kale and cook for 5-10 minutes.

7.   Serve!

Nutrition (Per Serving)

Calories: 121

Fat: 8g

Carbohydrates: 5g

Protein: 4g

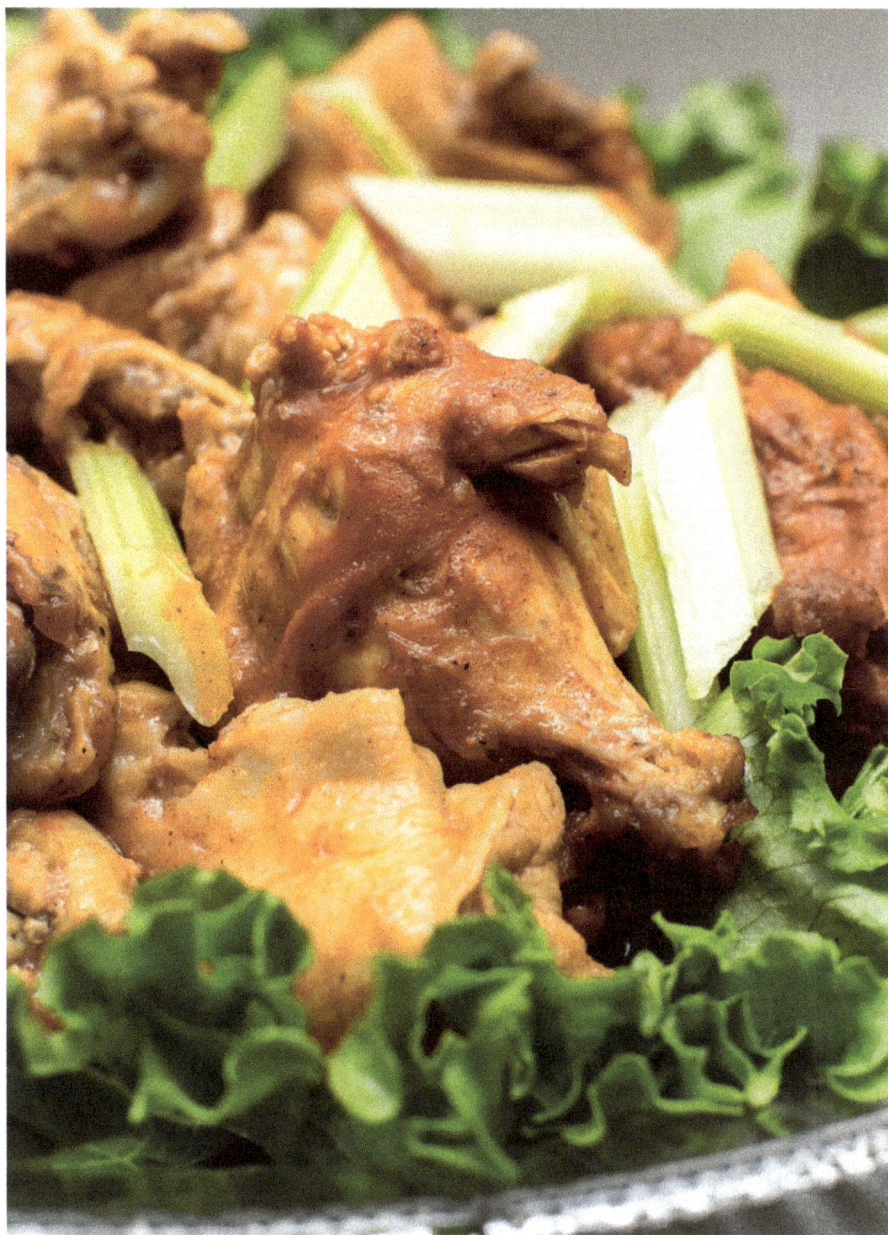

Acorn Squash with Mango Chutney

Serving: 4

Prep Time: 10 minutes

Cook Time: 3 hours 10 minutes

Ingredients:

1 large acorn squash

¼ cup mango chutney

¼ cup flaked coconut

Salt and pepper as needed

How To:

1.   Cut the squash into quarters and remove the seeds, discard the pulp.

2.   Spray your cooker with olive oil.

3.   Transfer the squash to the Slow Cooker and place lid.

4.   Take a bowl and add coconut and chutney, mix well and

divide the mixture into the center of the Squash.

5.   Season well.

6.   Place lid on top and cook on LOW for 2-3 hours.

7. Enjoy!

Nutrition (Per Serving)

Calories: 226

Fat: 6g

Carbohydrates: 24g

Protein: 17g

Amazing and Healthy Granola Bowl

Serving: 6

Prep Time: 5 minutes

Cook Time: 25 minutes

Ingredients:

1-ounce Porridge oats

2 teaspoons maple syrup

Cooking spray as needed

4 medium bananas

4 pots of Caramel

Layered Fromage Frais

5-ounce fresh fruit salad, such as strawberries, blueberries, and raspberries

¼ ounce pumpkin seeds

¼ ounce sunflower seeds

¼ ounce dry chia seeds

¼ ounce desiccated coconut

How To:

1.   Preheat your oven to 300 degrees F.

2.   Take a baking tray and line with baking paper.

3.   Take an outsized bowl and add oats, syrup, and seeds.

4.   Spread mix on a baking tray.

5.   Spray copra oil on top and bake for 20 minutes, ensuring to stay stirring from time to time.

6.   Sprinkle coconut after the primary quarter-hour.

7.   Remove from oven and let it cool.

8.   Take a bowl and layer sliced bananas on top of the Fromage Fraise.

9.   Spread the cooled granola mix on top and serve with a topping of berries.

10.   Enjoy!

Nutrition (Per Serving)

Calories: 446

Fat: 29g

Carbohydrates: 37g

Protein: 13g

Cinnamon and Pumpkin Porridge Medley

Serving: 2

Prep Time: 10 minutes

Cook Time: 15 minutes

Ingredients:

1 cup unsweetened almond/coconut milk

1 cup of water

1 cup uncooked quinoa

½ cup pumpkin puree

1 teaspoon ground cinnamon

2 tablespoons ground flaxseed meal

Juice of 1 lemon

How To:

1.   Take a pot and place it over medium-high heat.

2.   Whisk in water, almond milk and convey the combination to a boil.

3.   Stir in quinoa, cinnamon, and pumpkin.

4.   Reduce heat to low and simmer for 10 minutes until the liquid has evaporated.

5.   Remove from the warmth and stir in flaxseed meal.

6.   Transfer porridge to small bowls.

7.   Sprinkle juice and add pumpkin seeds on top.

8.   Serve and enjoy!

Nutrition (Per Serving)

Calories: 245

Fat: 1g

Carbohydrates: 59g

Protein: 4g

Quinoa and Date Bowl

Serving: 2

Prep Time: 10 minutes

Cook Time: 15 minutes

Ingredients:

1 date, pitted and chopped finely

½ cup red quinoa, dried

1 cup unsweetened almond milk

1/8 teaspoon vanilla extract

¼ cup fresh strawberries, hulled and sliced 1/8 teaspoon ground cinnamon

How To:

1.   Take a pan and place it over low heat.

2.   Add quinoa, almond milk, cinnamon, vanilla, and cook for about quarter-hour, ensuring to stay stirring from time to time.

3. Garnish with strawberries and enjoy!

Nutrition (Per Serving)

Calories: 195

Fat: 4.4g

Carbohydrates: 32g

Protein: 7g

Crispy Tofu

Serving: 8

Prep Time: 5 minutes

Cook Time: 20-30 minutes

Ingredients:

1-pound extra-firm tofu, drained and sliced

2 tablespoons olive oil

1 cup almond meal

1 tablespoons yeast

½ teaspoon onion powder ½ teaspoon garlic powder ½ teaspoon oregano

How To:

1.   Add all ingredients except tofu and vegetable oil during a shallow bowl.

2.   Mix well.

3.   Preheat your oven to 400 degrees F.

4.   during a wide bowl, add the almond meal and blend well.

5.	Brush tofu with vegetable oil, read the combination and coat well.

6.	Line a baking sheet with parchment paper.

7.	Transfer coated tofu to the baking sheet.

8.	Bake for 20-30 minutes, ensuring to flip once until golden brown.

9.	Serve and enjoy!

Nutrition (Per Serving)

Calories: 282

Fat: 20g

Carbohydrates: 9g

Protein: 12g

Hearty Pumpkin Oats

Serving: 3

Prep Time: 5 minutes

Cook Time: 8 minutes

Ingredients:

1 cup quick-cooking rolled oats

¾ cup almond milk

½ cup canned pumpkin puree

¼ teaspoon pumpkin pie spice

1 teaspoon ground cinnamon

How To:

1.   Take a secure microwave bowl and add oats, almond milk, and microwave on high for 1-2 minutes.

2.   Add more almond milk if needed to realize your required consistency.

3.   Cook for 30 seconds more.

4.   Stir in pumpkin puree, pie spice, ground cinnamon.

5.   Heat gently and enjoy!

Nutrition (Per Serving)

Calories: 229

Fat: 4g

Carbohydrates: 38g

Protein:10g

Wholesome Pumpkin Pie Oatmeal

Serving: 2

Prep Time: 10 minutes

Cook Time: 10 minutes

Smart Points: 6

Ingredients:

½ cup canned pumpkin, low sodium

Mashed banana as needed

¾ cup unsweetened almond milk

½ teaspoon pumpkin pie spice

1 cup oats

How To:

1.   Mash banana employing a fork and blend within the remaining ingredients (except oats) and blend well.

2.   Add oats and finely stir.

3.   Transfer mixture to a pot and let the oats cook until it's absorbed the liquid and is tender.

4.   Serve and enjoy!

Nutrition (Per Serving)

Calories: 264

Fat: 4g

Carbohydrates: 52g

Protein: 7g

Power-Packed Oatmeal

Serving: 2

Prep Time: 10-15 minutes

Cook Time: 5 minutes

Ingredients:

¼ cup quick-cooking oats

¼ cup almond milk

2 tablespoons low fat Greek yogurt

¼ banana, mashed

2-1/4 tablespoons flaxseed meal

How To:

1.   Whisk altogether of the ingredients during a bowl.

2.   Transfer the bowl to your fridge and let it refrigerate for quarter-hour.

3.   Serve and enjoy!

Nutrition (Per Serving)

Calories:

Fat: 11g

Carbohydrates: 27g

Protein: 10g

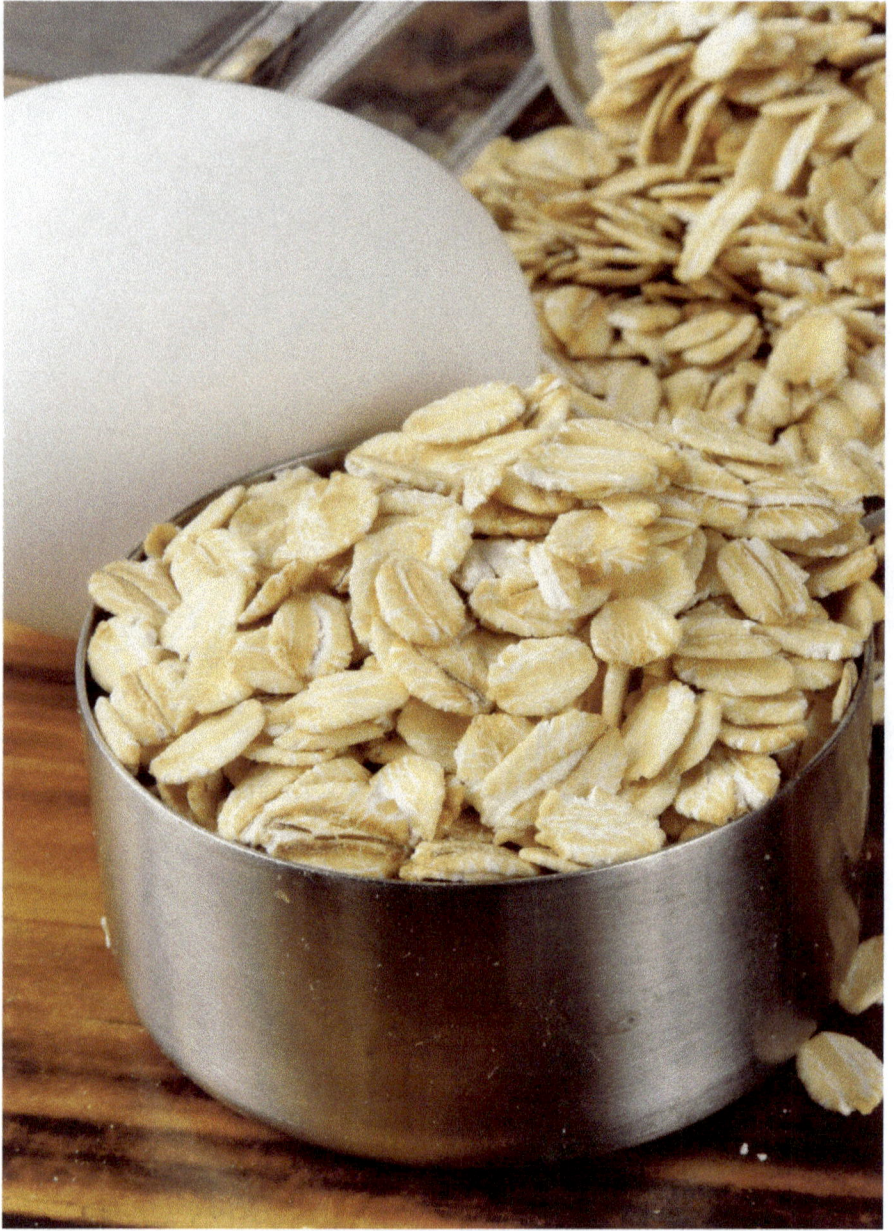

Saucy Garlic Greens

Serving: 4

Prep Time: 5 minutes

Cook Time: 20 minutes

Ingredients:

1 bunch of leafy greens Sauce

½ cup cashews soaked in water for 10 minutes ¼ cup water

1 tablespoon lemon juice

1 teaspoon coconut aminos

1 clove peeled whole clove

1/8 teaspoon of flavored vinegar

How To:

1.   Make the sauce by draining and discarding the soaking water from your cashews and add the cashews to a blender.

2.   Add water, juice, flavored vinegar, coconut aminos, garlic.

3.   Blitz until you've got a smooth cream and transfer to bowl.

4.   Add ½ cup of water to the pot.

5.   Place the steamer basket to the pot and add the greens within the basket.

6.   Lock the lid and steam for 1 minute.

7.   Quick-release the pressure.

8.   Transfer the steamed greens to strainer and extract excess water.

9.   Place the greens into a bowl.

10.   Add lemon aioli and toss.

11.   Enjoy!

Nutrition (Per Serving)

Calories: 77

Fat: 5g

Carbohydrates: 0g

Protein: 2g

Garden Salad

Serving: 6

Prep Time: 5 minutes

Cook Time: 20 minutes

Ingredients:

1-pound raw peanuts in shell

1 bay leaf

2 medium-sized chopped up tomatoes

½ cup diced up green pepper

½ cup diced up sweet onion

¼ cup finely diced hot pepper

¼ cup diced up celery

2 tablespoons olive oil

¾ teaspoon flavored vinegar

¼ teaspoon freshly ground black pepper

How To:

1.   Boil your peanuts for 1 minute and rinse them.

2.   The skins are going to be soft, so discard the skin.

3.   Add 2 cups of water to the moment Pot.

4.   Add herb and peanuts.

5.   Lock the lid and cook on high for 20 minutes.

6.   Drain the water.

7.   Take an outsized bowl and add the peanuts, diced up vegetables.

8.   Whisk in vegetable oil, juice, pepper in another bowl.

9.   Pour the mixture over the salad and blend.

10.   Enjoy!

Nutrition (Per Serving)

Calories: 140

Fat: 4g

Carbohydrates: 24g

Protein: 5g

Spicy Cabbage Dish

Serving: 4

Prep Time: 10 minutes

Cooking Time: 4 hours

Ingredients:

2 yellow onions, chopped

10 cups red cabbage, shredded

1 cup plums, pitted and chopped

1 teaspoon cinnamon powder

1 garlic clove, minced

1 teaspoon cumin seeds

¼ teaspoon cloves, ground

2 tablespoons red wine vinegar

1 teaspoon coriander seeds

½ cup water

How To:

1.   Add cabbage, onion, plums, garlic, cumin, cinnamon, cloves, vinegar, coriander and water to your Slow Cooker.

2.   Stir well.

3.   Place lid and cook on LOW for 4 hours.

4.   Divide between serving platters.

5.   Enjoy!

Nutrition (Per Serving)

Calories: 197

Fat: 1g

Carbohydrates: 14g

Protein: 3g

Extreme Balsamic Chicken

Serving: 4

Prep Time: 10 minutes

Cook Time: 35 minutes

Ingredients:

3 boneless chicken breasts, skinless

Sunflower seeds to taste

¼ cup almond flour

2/3 cups low-fat chicken broth

1 ½ teaspoons arrowroot

½ cup low sugar raspberry preserve

1 ½ tablespoons balsamic vinegar

How To:

1.   Cut pigeon breast into bite-sized pieces and season them with seeds.

2.   Dredge the chicken pieces in flour and shake off any excess.

3. Take a non-stick skillet and place it over medium heat.

4. Add chicken to the skillet and cook for quarter-hour , ensuring to show them half-way through.

5. Remove chicken and transfer to platter.

6. Add arrowroot, broth, raspberry preserve to the skillet and stir.

7. Stir in balsamic vinegar and reduce heat to low, stir-cook for a couple of minutes.

8. Transfer the chicken back to the sauce and cook for quarter-hour more.

9. Serve and enjoy!

Nutrition (Per Serving)

Calories: 546

Fat: 35g

Carbohydrates: 11g

Protein: 44g

Enjoyable Spinach and Bean Medley

Serving: 4

Prep Time: 10 minutes

Cooking Time: 4 hours

Ingredients:

5 carrots, sliced

1 ½ cups great northern beans, dried

2 garlic cloves, minced

1 yellow onion, chopped

Pepper to taste

½ teaspoon oregano, dried

5 ounces baby spinach

4 ½ cups low sodium veggie stock

2 teaspoons lemon peel, grated

3 tablespoon lemon juice

How To:

1.   Add beans, onion, carrots, garlic, oregano and stock to your Slow Cooker.

2.   Stir well.

3.   Place lid and cook on HIGH for 4 hours.

4.   Add spinach, juice and lemon rind.

5.   Stir and let it sit for five minutes.

6.   Divide between serving platters and enjoy!

Nutrition (Per Serving)

Calories: 219

Fat: 8g

Carbohydrates: 14g

Protein: 8g

Brown Butter Duck Breast

Serving: 3

Prep Time: 5 minutes

Cook Time: 25 minutes

Ingredients:

1 whole 6-ounce duck breast, skin on

Pepper to taste

1 head radicchio, 4 ounces, core removed ¼ cup unsalted butter

6 fresh sage leaves, sliced

How To:

1.   Pre-heat your oven to 400-degree F.

2.   Pat duck breast dry with towel.

3.   Season with pepper.

4.   Place duck breast in skillet and place it over medium heat, sear for 3-4 minutes all sides

5.   Turn breast over and transfer skillet to oven.

6.   Roast for 10 minutes (uncovered).

7.   Cut radicchio in half.

8.   Remove and discard the woody white core and thinly slice the leaves.

9.   Keep them on the side.

10.   Remove skillet from oven.

11.   Transfer duck breast, fat side up to chopping board and let it rest.

12.   Re-heat your skillet over medium heat.

13. Add unsalted butter, sage and cook for 3-4 minutes.

14.   Cut duck into 6 equal slices.

15.   Divide radicchio between 2 plates, top with slices of duck breast and drizzle browned butter and sage.

16.   Enjoy!

Nutrition (Per Serving)

Calories: 393

Fat: 33g

Carbohydrates: 2g

Protein: 22g

Generous Garlic Bread Stick

Serving: 8 breadsticks

Prep Time: 15 minutes

Cooking Time: 15 minutes

Ingredients:

¼ cup almond butter, softened

1 teaspoon garlic powder

2 cups almond flour

½ tablespoon baking powder

1 tablespoon Psyllium husk powder

¼ teaspoon sunflower seeds

3 tablespoons almond butter, melted

1 egg

¼ cup boiling water

How To:

1.   Pre-heat your oven to 400 degrees F.

2.   Line baking sheet with parchment paper and keep it on the side.

3.   Beat almond butter with garlic powder and keep it on the side.

4.   Add almond flour, leaven, husk, sunflower seeds during a bowl and blend in almond butter and egg, mix well.

5.   Pour boiling water within the mix and stir until you've got a pleasant dough.

6.   Divide the dough into 8 balls and roll into breadsticks.

7.   Place on baking sheet and bake for quarter-hour.

8.   Brush each persist with garlic almond butter and bake for five minutes more.

9.   Serve and enjoy!

Nutrition (Per Serving)

Total Carbs: 7g

Fiber: 2g

Protein: 7g

Fat: 24g

Cauliflower Bread Stick

Serving: 5 breadsticks

Prep Time: 10 minutes

Cooking Time: 48 minutes

Ingredients:

1 cup cashew cheese/ kite ricotta cheese

1 tablespoon organic almond butter

1 whole egg

½ teaspoon Italian seasoning

¼ teaspoon red pepper flakes

1/8 teaspoon kosher sunflower seeds

2 cups cauliflower rice, cooked for 3 minutes in microwave

3 teaspoons garlic, minced

Parmesan cheese, grated

How To:

1.   Pre-heat your oven to 350 degrees F.

2.   Add almond butter during a small pan and melt over low heat

3.   Add red pepper flakes, garlic to the almond butter and cook for 2-3 minutes.

4.   Add garlic and almond butter mix to the bowl with cooked cauliflower and add the Italian seasoning.

5.   Season with sunflower seeds and blend, refrigerate for 10 minutes.

6.   Add cheese and eggs to the bowl and blend.

7.   Place a layer of parchment paper at rock bottom of a 9 x 9 baking dish and grease with cooking spray, add egg and mozzarella cheese mix to the cauliflower mix.

8.   Add mix to the pan and smooth to a skinny layer with the palms of your hand.

9.   Bake for half-hour , remove from oven and top with few shakes of parmesan and mozzarella.

10.   Cook for 8 minutes more.

11.   Enjoy!

Nutrition (Per Serving)

Total Carbs: 11.5g

Fiber: 2g

Protein: 10.7g

Fat: 20g

Bacon and Chicken Garlic Wrap

Serving: 4

Prep Time: 15 minutes

Cook Time: 10 minutes

Ingredients:

1 chicken fillet, cut into small cubes

8-9 thin slices bacon, cut to fit cubes

6 garlic cloves, minced

How To:

1.   Pre-heat your oven to 400 degrees F.

2.   Line a baking tray with aluminum foil .

3.   Add minced garlic to a bowl and rub each chicken piece with it.

4.   Wrap a bacon piece around each garlic chicken bite.

5.   Secure with toothpick.

6.   Transfer bites to baking sheet, keeping a touch little bit of space between them.

7. Bake for about 15-20 minutes until crispy.

8. Serve and enjoy!

Nutrition (Per Serving)

Calories: 260

Fat: 19g

Carbohydrates: 5g

Protein: 22g

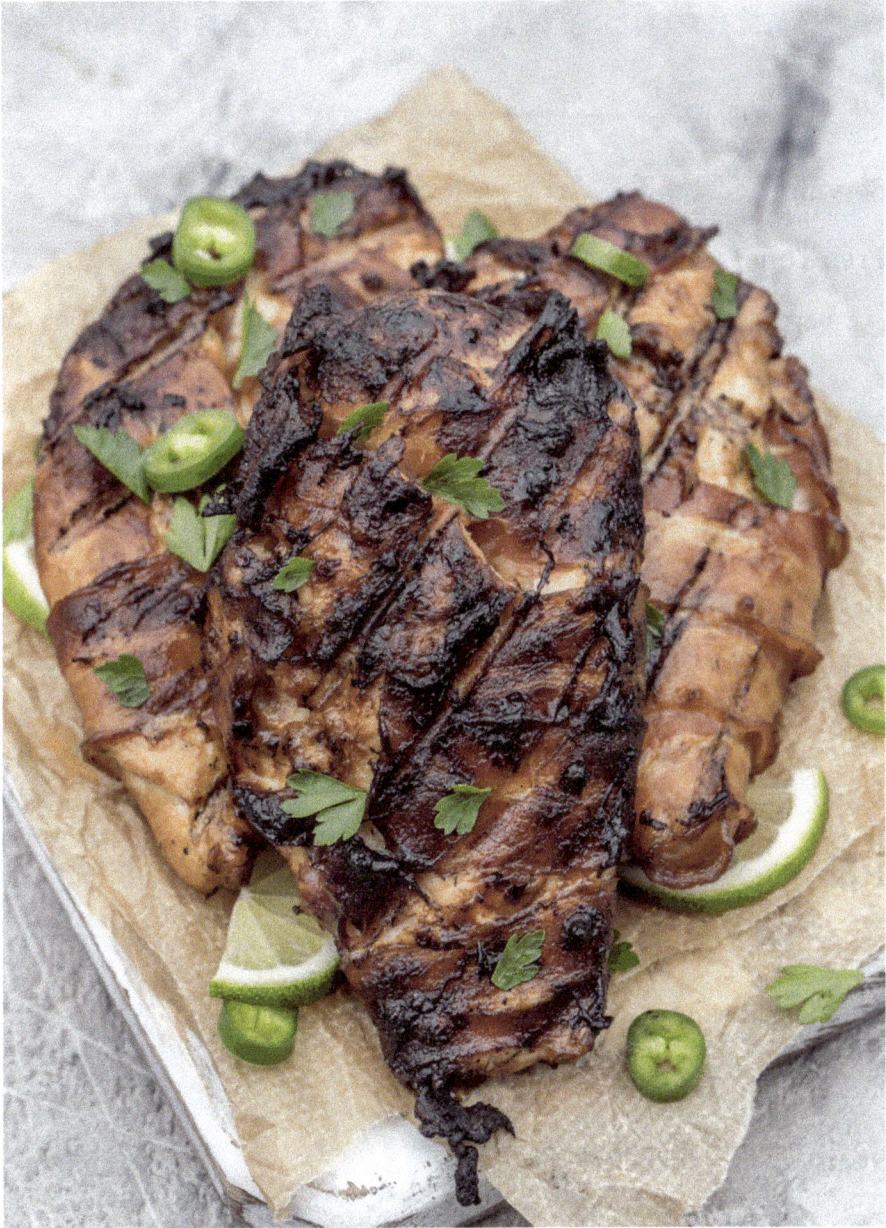

Portuguese Kale and Sausage Soup

Serving: 4

Prep Time: 10 minutes

Cook Time: 35 minutes

Ingredients:

1 yellow onion, chopped

16 ounces sausage, chopped

3 sweet potatoes, chopped

4cups chicken stock1 pound kale, chopped pepper as needed

How To:

1.   Take a pot and place it over medium heat.

2.   Add sausage and brown each side.

3.   Transfer to bowl.

4.   Heat pot again over medium heat.

5.   Add onion and stir for five minutes.

6.   Add stock, sweet potatoes, stir and convey to a simmer.

7.   Cook for 20 minutes.

8.   Use an immersion blender to blend.

9.   Add kale and pepper and simmer for two minutes over low heat.

10.   Ladle soup to bowls and top with sausage with pieces.

11.   Serve and enjoy!

Nutrition (Per Serving)

Calories: 200

Fat: 2g

Carbohydrates: 6g

Protein:8g

Dazzling Pizza Soup

Serving: 6

Prep Time: 5 minutes

Cook Time: 30 minutes

Ingredients:

12 ounces chicken meat, sliced

4 ounces uncured pepperoni

1 can 25 ounces marinara

1 can 14.5 ounces fire roasted tomatoes

1 large onion, diced

15 ounces mushrooms, sliced

1 can 3 ounce sliced black olives

tablespoon dried oregano

1 teaspoon garlic powder

½ teaspoon salt

How To:

1.   Take large sized saucepan and add within the peperoni, chicken meat, marinara, onions, tomatoes, mushroom, oregano, olives, salt and garlic powder.

2.   Cook the mixture for half-hour over medium level heat and soften the mushroom and onions.

3.   Serve hot.

Nutrition (Per Serving)

Calories: 90

Fat: 2g

Carbohydrates: 17g

Protein: 3g

Mesmerizing Lentil Soup

Serving: 4

Prep Time: 10 minutes

Cooking Time: 8 hours

Ingredients:

1 pound dried lentils, soaked overnight and rinsed carrots, peeled and chopped

1 celery stalk, chopped

1 onion, chopped

6 cups vegetables broth

1 ½ teaspoons garlic powder

1 teaspoon ground cumin

1 teaspoon smoked paprika

1 teaspoon dried thyme

¼ teaspoon liquid smoke

¼ teaspoon salt

¼ teaspoon ground pepper

How To:

1.　　Add listed ingredients to Slow Cooker and stir well.

2.　　Place lid and cook for 8 hours on LOW.

3.　　Stir and serve.

4.　　Enjoy!

Nutrition (Per Serving)

Calories: 307

Fat: 1g

Carbohydrates: 56g

Protein: 20g

Organically Healthy Chicken Soup

Serving: 4

Prep Time: 10 minutes

Cook Time: 12-15 minutes

Ingredients:

cans (14 ounces each) low sodium chicken broth 2 cups water

1 cup twisted spaghetti

¼ teaspoon pepper

cups mixed vegetables (such as broccoli, carrots etc.)

1 and ½ cups chicken, cooked and cubed

1 tablespoon fresh basil, snipped

¼ cup parmesan, finely shredded

How To:

1. Take a Dutch Oven and add broth, water, pepper and bring the mixture to a boil. 2. Gently stir in pasta and wait until the mixture reaches boiling point again,

2.   Lower down the heat and let the mixture simmer for 5 minutes (covered).

3.   Remove lid and stir in the vegetables, return the mixture boil and lower down heat once again.

4.   Cover and let it simmer over low heat for 5-8 minutes until the pasta and veggies and tender and cooked.

5.   Stir in cooked chicken and garnish with basil.

6.   Serve with a topping of parmesan.

7.   Enjoy!

Nutrition Values (Per Serving)

Calories: 400

Fat: 9g

Carbohydrates: 37g

Protein: 45g

Potato and Asparagus Bisque

Serving: 4

Prep Time: 5 minutes

Cook Time: 6 minutes

Ingredients:

1 ½ pound asparagus

2 pounds sweet potatoes

cups vegetable broth

1 large sized onion

8 cloves garlic

2 tablespoons dried dill

2 tablespoons flavored vinegar

3-4 cups almond milk

4 tablespoons Dijon mustard

4 tablespoons yeast

How To:

1.   Add the listed ingredients (except milk, mustard and yeast) to your pot.

2.   Lock the lid and cook on HIGH pressure for 6 minutes.

3.   Release the pressure naturally.

4.   Open the lid and add almond milk, yeast and mustard.

5.   Puree using immersion blender.

6.   Serve over rice.

7.   Enjoy!

Nutrition (Per Serving)

Calories: 430

Fat: 12g

Carbohydrates: 77g

Protein: 6g

Cabbage and Leek Soup

Serving: 4

Prep Time: 10 minutes

Cook Time: 25 minutes

Ingredients:

2 tablespoons coconut oil

½ head chopped up cabbage

3-4 diced ribs celery

2-3 carefully cleaned and chopped leeks

1 diced bell pepper

2-3 diced carrots

2/3 cloves minced garlic

4 cups chicken broth

1 teaspoon Italian seasoning

1 teaspoon Creole seasoning

Black pepper as needed

2-3 cups mixed salad greens

How To:

1.	Set your pot to Sauté mode and add coconut oil.

2.	Allow the oil to heat up.

3.	Add the veggies (except salad greens) starting from the carrot, making sure to stir well after each vegetable addition.

4.	Make sure to add the garlic last.

5.	Season with Italian seasoning, black pepper and Creole seasoning.

6.	Add broth and lock the lid.

7.	Cook on SOUP mode for 20 minutes.

8.	Release the pressure naturally and add salad greens, stir well and allow to sit for a while.

9.	Allow for a few minutes to wilt the veggies.

10.	Season with a bit of flavored vinegar and pepper and enjoy!

Nutrition (Per Serving)

Calories: 32

Fat: 0g

Carbohydrates: 4g

Protein: 2g

Onion Soup

Serving: 4

Prep Time: 10 minutes

Cook Time: 3 hours

Ingredients:

2 tablespoons avocado oil

yellow onions, cut into halved and sliced Black pepper to taste 5 cups beef stock

3 thyme sprigs

1 tablespoon tomato paste

How To:

1.   Take a pot and place it over medium high heat.

2.   Add onion and thyme and stir.

3.   Reduce heat to low and cook for 30 minutes.

4.   Uncover pot and cook onions for 1 hour and 30 minutes more, stirring often.

5.   Add tomato paste, stock and stir.

6.   Simmer for 1 hour more.

7.   Ladle soup into bowls and enjoy!

Nutrition (Per Serving)

Calories: 200

Fat: 4g

Carbohydrates: 6g

Protein: 8g

Carrot, Ginger and Turmeric Soup

Serving: 4

Prep Time: 15 minutes

Cook Time: 40 minutes

Ingredients:

cups chicken broth

¼ cup full fat coconut milk, unsweetened ¾ pound carrots, peeled and chopped 1 teaspoon turmeric, ground

2 teaspoons ginger, grated

1 yellow onion, chopped

2 garlic cloves, peeled

Pinch of pepper

How To:

1.   Take a stockpot and add all the ingredients except coconut milk into it.

2.   Place stockpot over medium heat.

3.   Bring to a boil.

4.   Reduce heat to simmer for 40 minutes.

5.   Remove the bay leaf.

6.   Blend the soup until smooth by using an immersion blender.

7.   Add the coconut milk and stir.

8.   Serve immediately and enjoy!

Nutrition (Per Serving)

Calories: 79

Fat: 4g

Carbohydrates: 7g

Protein: 4g

Offbeat Squash Soup

Serving: 4

Prep Time: 10 minutes

Cook Time: 50 minutes

Ingredients:

1 butternut squash, cut in halve lengthwise and deseeded

14 ounces coconut milk

Pinch of salt

Black pepper to taste

Handful of parsley, chopped

Pinch of nutmeg, ground

How To:

1.   Add butternut squash halves on a lined baking sheet.

2.   Place in oven and bake for 45 minutes at 350 degrees F.

3.   Leave squash to cool down and scoop out the flesh to a pot.

4.   Add half of the coconut milk to the pot and blend using immersion blender.

5.   Heat soup over medium-low heat and add remaining coconut milk.

6.   Add a pinch of salt, black pepper to taste.

7.   Add nutmeg, parsley and blend using an immersion blender once again for a few seconds.

8.   Cook for 4 minutes.

9.   Serve and enjoy!

Nutrition (Per Serving)

Calories: 144

Fat: 10g

Carbohydrates: 7g

Protein: 2g

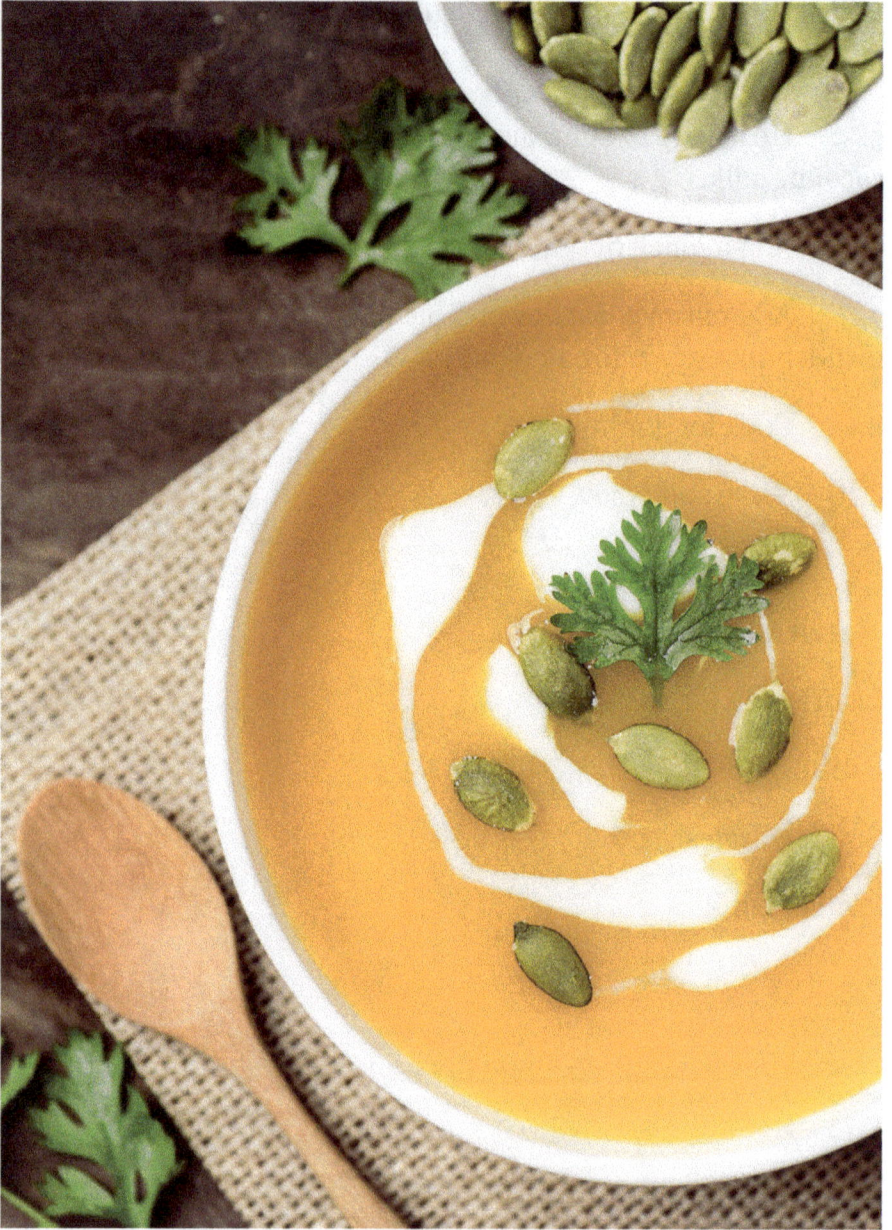

www.ingramcontent.com/pod-product-compliance
Lightning Source LLC
Chambersburg PA
CBHW050752030426
42336CB00012B/1782